Chitosan

by
William J. Hennen, Ph.D.

Woodland Publishing Inc.
P.O. Box 160
Pleasant Grove, UT 84062

TABLE OF CONTENTS

PREVIEW

The lifestyles of western cultures have been determined to be major contributing factors in diseases such as heart disease, diabetes and cancer. The most commonly cited factors are inadequate fiber intake, excessive consumption of fats, and a lack of exercise. Educational efforts have resulted in an increase in involvement in various exercise regimines. The consumption of fats, however, continues to increase in spite of the dire warnings that have been publicized. A reduction of fat intake, from an average of 40 percent of the diet to less than 25 percent could have dramatic effects on the health and well-being of the population as a whole. Intake of fiberous foods reduces fat consumption generally through the bulking action of the fibers which leads to a feelings of fullness. Some fibers have an ability to entrap fats in their gelatinous matrix and prevent their absorption. The most effective fiber for preventing fat absorption is chitosan. Chitosan's fat entrapment properties can be enhanced by combination with ascorbic acid and other dietary ingredients. Fat entrapment by chitosan has been shown in animals and can be readily demonstrated. The use of chitosan in nummerous environmental, agricultual, biomedical, and health-related areas is well documented. Chitosan has been found to be safe for oral consumption.

INTRODUCTION

Stated simply, Chitosan is an extraordinary fat binder. Chemically speaking, Chitosan is an amino polysaccharide that has the ability to "bind" lipids in the stomach before they are absorbed through the digestive system into the bloodstream. The presence of fats in the blood can raise cholesterol levels, contribute to cardiovascular disease and cancer, and most importantly, promote obesity.

Not only does chitosan attract and inhibit fats, it offers an array of other desirable physiological benefits that can foster optimal health and longevity. In an era where everyone is interested in decreasing their fat intake, Chitosan can act as a remarkable supplement. When taken prior to eating or during a meal, it can significantly reduce the body's absorption of dietary fats.

Of equal significance is the fact that when Chitosan is combined with other compounds such as citric acid, ascorbic acid and phytochemicals called indoles, its action is enhanced, making it far more valuable as both a fat binder and dietary health aid. Fat is responsible for more of our health "ills" than any other single substance. Chitosan provides a simple and safe complement to smart eating and exercise to control lipid levels.

FEARING FATS: There's Plenty of Cause

Overview

A wealth of scientific evidence now exists which should have turned each and everyone of us into a fat "phobic."[1a-e] In other words, virtually every health expert agrees that a high fat diet is directly linked to cardiovascular disease, various types of cancer and premature death.

It's no secret that excess dietary fat poses a tremendous health risk. The United States National Institutes of Health, the World Health Organization and many other scientific institutes have confirmed the frightening hazards of fat. Health proponents generally concur that excess fat can significantly shorten one's lifespan.

More than 10,000 medical papers are published every year dealing with obesity and cardiovascular disease, two of the most insidious killers of Americans. Western eating habits, which promote fatty, salty, sugary foods, have created massive widespread disease and tremendous suffering.

Studies have shown that fat is the macronutrient associated with overeating and obesity.[2] In spite of this finding we are eating more fat and becoming fatter. The average absolute fat intake has increased from 81 to 83 grams per day over the last ten years.[3] Our obsession with fatty foods has exacted an enormous toll in the form of rampant obesity, clogged arteries, hypertension, heart attack, stroke, breast cancer, etc. Many of us remain oblivious to the fat gram count of foods we routinely pop into our mouths, unaware that one fast food entree may contain more fat grams than one should consume in one given day. Take a good look at the following list of foods which have been assessed for fat content.

• BACON CHEESEBURGER/HARDEE'S	39
• BURRITO SUPREME/TACO BELL	22
• HAMBURGER DELUXE/WENDY'S	21
• QUARTER POUNDER WITH CHEESE/MCDONALD'S	28
• SAUSAGE BISCUIT WITH EGG/MCDONALD'S	33
• POPCORN CHICKEN/KFC	45
• WHOPPER/BURGER KING	36

TABLE 1. *Total fat grams in single servings.*[4]

Fast food has become a 20th-century sensation which continues to boom and expand throughout our society. Many of us literally exist on fast food, which is frequently also "fat" food. It's no wonder so many of us "battle the bulge", and have skyrocketing cholesterol counts. Our love affair with greasy, fried, rich, creamy foods has burdened our bodies with the dilemma of excess fat "baggage," resulting in phenomenal amounts of money being spent on weight loss programs. Worse still, thousands of Americans are dying before their time or living extremely compromised lives only because they ingest too much fat. Why is this? The bottom line is that fats taste good![5]

Many of us were raised on seemingly innocuous foods that are loaded with fat. Some of these include:

macaroni and cheese	*battered fish sticks*	*hot dogs*
cheese-filled casseroles	*pepperoni pizza*	*burritos*

| pancakes, waffles | doughnuts | pies and pastries |
| ice cream | candy bars | ramen soup |

Fat is also a major ingredient in most of the snack food we constantly nibble on, including chips, crackers, cookies, and nuts.

Check ingredient labels to find the fat gram content of most snack foods. You'll be surprised to find out just how fatty these foods are. Even a healthy sounding food like a "bran muffin" can contain 36 grams of fat! No wonder they stay so "moist".

In addition to the above foods, fat can add wonderful flavor to breads, vegetables and the like, and is usually used liberally in the form of butter, sour cream, whipping cream, melted cheese, cream cheese spreads, dips, cream sauces, and gravies. Fruits can also be high in fats. Did you know that one avocado has 30 grams of fat? One half cup of peanuts contains 35 grams of fat and only one glazed doughnut has 13 grams of fat.

The majority of research points to fat as a much more dangerous culprit than anyone might have imagined. Saturated fats such as lard, palm, coconut oil, and beef tallow are particularly menacing. Research scientists have found over and over again that fats can contribute to the growth of tumors in animal studies.[6]

The National Research Council of the National Academy of Sciences reported that even a relatively small amount of extra body fat increases the risk of certain diseases for women and may compromise their longevity.[7] Even being mildly overweight may be much more risky than anyone previously assumed.[8]

The Relationship between Breast Cancer, Fats, Fiber And Indoles

Dr. Leonard Cohen, of the Dana Institute of the American Health Foundation at Naylor, believes that pre-cancerous lesions found in breast tissue will develop into cancer only if they are stimulated by certain agents such as fat.[9]

Women increase their risk of developing breast cancer when they consume a diet high in fat and animal protein and low in fiber, vegetables and fruits.

When women put on weight, they have a tendency to create more estrogen since adipose tissue produces estrogen. Certain forms of estrogen, the so-called "bad estrogens" can act as carcinogens and are anything but desirable.[10] High or unbalanced estrogen levels stimulate concerous tissue in the breast. Obesity is also associated with increased breast cancer mortality.[11]

The three most important ways to inhibit "bad" estrogen from inducing breast cancer are:

1. Maintain an ideal body weight.

2. Eat a diet high in fiber and low in fat (fiber helps to sweep excess estrogen from the bowel so it does not "recycle").

3. Consume enough cruciferous vegetables (broccoli, cabbage, cauliflower, Brussels sprouts, kale, radishes, watercress etc.) so that adequate amounts of dietary indole-3-carbinol enter the system.[12]

Indoles are phytonutrients which help us balance our estrogen levels and reduce the levels of "bad estrogen" present. When combined with a low-fat, high-fiber diet, indoles can provide the body with significant metabolic protection against breast cancer.

The Relationship between Cervical, Uterine and Endometrial Cancers and Lipids

The cascade between a high-fat, low-fiber diet, obesity, and dangerous estrogen levels also plays a role in the development of cervical, uterine, and endometrial cancers.[13] It has been reported by the National Academy of Science that "diet is responsible for 60 percent or more of all cancer in women. The most important dietary change you can make to protect against these diseases is to reduce dietary fat to less that 30 percent of total calories, preferably to less than 25 percent."[14]

Prostate Cancer And Fat

The incidence of prostate cancer has also been linked to fat consumption for all ethnic groups.[15, 16] Animal studies have shown that the promotional effects of a high-fat diet on prostate cancer can be found even in the mother's preconceptual diet and the early adolecent diet.[17] Conversely, mice fed a low-fat diet demonstrated dramatic drops in prostate tumor growth rates.[18]

Colo-rectal Cancer and Fat

Dietary fat intake has been closely related to the incidence of colon cancer in this country.[19, 20] "Diet is probably the major determinant of the risk of colo-rectal cancer; there is evidence that fruit and vegetables and fiber reduce risk and that meat and animal fat increase risk[.]"[20] Due to the action of intestinal microflora, undigested meats and fats can be chemically altered to form carcinogenic chemicals chich can damage the lining of the colon and promote the formation of cell mutations.[21] Again the case for a high-fiber, low-saturated-fat diet is evident.

Cardiovascular Disease (CVD) and Fat Consumption

Overview

If we let ourselves become obese, we are much more prone to developing heart disease, high blood pressure, stroke, diabetes and several forms of cancer. Cardiovascular disease (CVD) or coronary heart disease (CHD) is the leading cause of death and disease in our country—512,000 people die of heart attacks every year (American Heart Assoc. 1995, Statistical Report).

Blood cholesterol levels are the primary indicators of one's risk of CHD. It is not surprising then that ten of the twelve points listed by the National Heart Foundation of Australia relating diet and coronary heart disease involved cholesterol levels.[22] The take-home message was to eat a high-fiber, low-saturated-fat diet, and increase the amounts of essential fatty acids in our diets.

HDL and LDL Cholesterol

There are both "good" and "bad" forms of cholesterol. The "good" form of cholesterol is found in the form of high-density lipoproteins (HDLs). The 'bad" forms of cholesterol are the low-density lipoproteins (LDLs).

The types of fats we eat influence how much and what type of cholesterol we make. Saturated fats are particularly good at raising low-density lipoprotein or LDL cholesterol. The more of this type of cholesterol we have floating around in our bloodstream, the greater our risk of developing atherosclerosis, heart attack and stroke. The more HDL cholesterol we have (high-density lipoproteins) the lower our risk of coronary heart disease.

---

a) Elevated total blood cholesterol levels greater than 200 mg per deciliter
b) Elevated LDL cholesterol levels greater than 130 mg per deciliter
c) HDL cholesterol levels that create a ratio of total cholesterol to HDL cholesterol greater than 4.5 to 1
d) Obesity
e) Fat stores which accumulate above the waist

TABLE 2. *Cholesterol factors that increase the risk of developing heart disease.*

The liver is constantly trying to clear out the bad cholesterol by dumping it into the intestines. If we have sufficient amounts of the right kinds of fiber in our diet, our bodies dispose of cholesterol waste rather than reabsorbing it back into the blood stream. If we don't eat sufficient amounts of the right kinds of fiber, the cholesterol waste is reabsorbed and adds to the toxic stress on the body—especially the liver.

The obesity factor is emerging as much more important than previously thought.[23, 24] New findings strongly suggest that even a relatively small amount of excess weight (between 10 and 20 pounds) can predispose one to the development of heart disease.[25]

Boosting Fiber Consumption To Prevent CVD

"Dietary fiber reduces blood fat and blood pressure."[26] While most of us know how important it is to reduce the amount of fat we consume, many of us remain oblivious to the very profound role that fiber plays in helping to keep our arteries clear, preventing obesity and expediting elimination of toxins from the bowel. [27]

Ideally, a decrease in dietary fats combined with an increase in fiber and exercise comprise the winning prescription for preventing CHD.[28, 29] Coronary heart disease is an insidious killer which can go undetected until it's too late.

Diabetes and Body Fat

A recent examination of diabetes in the U.S. revealed some startling facts:[30]

a) Over 13 million people in the United States have diabetes.
b) Women represent about 60 percent of all new cases of diabetes.
c) Diabetes is more common among Native American, black, and Hispanic women than among white women.
d) Women with diabetes are at greater risk for CHD.
e) Women with diabetes are at greater risk for developing endometrial cancer.

TABLE 3. *Diabetes in the United States*

The increased incidence of diabetes with age has long been known.[31] However, if one looks more closely, it is obesity, not age, that is the more directly related factor.[32] Becoming overweight is one of the most significant contributors to the development of adult-onset diabetes.[33, 34, 35] Biological mechanisms explaining how obesity leads to diabetes have been proposed.[36] But this is much less important than the fact that diabetes, like obesity and heart disease, is strongly affected by what we eat.[30] Again high-fat, low-fiber diets coupled with a sedentary lifestyle are a prescription for disaster. Is it any wonder then that diabetes, obesity and heart disease so often occur together in what has been called "generalized cardiovascular-metabolic disease"?[37, 38] Some individuals with non-insulin dependent diabetes (adult-onset diabetes) overcome this disorder just by losing excess weight, a fact which highlights once again the perils of those extra pounds.

Aches and Pains

The dietary factors that are considered to influence the formation of cholesterol gallstones include high intake of cholesterol and fat and low intake of fiber.[39] Similarly our high-fat low fiber diets which make us obese lead to osteoarthritis.[40] The extra weight we carry puts extra strain on our joints, can cause osteoarthritis, and is one of the reasons we avoid exercise— it definitely hurts! Our western eating habits are giving us some very real pains.

OBESITY: A 20th-Century Plague

Overview

Our modern, fast-paced, high stress, sedentary lifestyle with over-abundant caloric intake is a prescription for obesity. Obesity is an especially critical problem for black women who have nearly twice the rate of obesity of white women.[41]

Culturally, being overweight is not looked on graciously, even by physicians.[42] There has been no end to the torture we have put ourselves through to be or at least look thin. From corsets to stomach stapling and liposuction to wiring our jaws shut, we've tried it all. So where are we today? The following are indicators of abundant obesity:

Research and public education efforts are in agreement that excessive dietary fat is the primary cause of adult obesity.[2, 46, 47] Despite the fact that food manufacturers have flooded the supermarkets with low-fat, artificially sweetened, "lite" products, we are fatter than ever before.

---

a) The overwhelming majority of all adults are unhappy with their appearance and fitness.
b) More of our children are obese today than ever before.
c) Two out of three people will regain the weight they lose on a diet program within one year.
d) 33 billion dollars is spent annually on weight-loss programs.
e) 33 percent of all adult Americans are over weight.

TABLE 4. *Obesity in the United States*

Is maintaining a healthy weight really that difficult? In its simplest form gaining or losing weight is a matter of the balance between energy in and energy out. This simplistic approach led to the early starvation diets. Unquestionably, these conventional very-low-calorie diet plans do not work. For most of us the first thing we lose is our sense of humor; then maybe some weight or possibly our self-esteem. The fact is, as most of us have regrettably discovered, that drastically reducing our calorie tally only serves to slow our metabolism and make us even more efficient at the business of storing and hoarding fat.

Since very-low-calorie diets didn't work alone, exercise was added to the regime. This also failed miserably because the first thing the body does when it is in a starvation mode is to burn off muscle mass so as to conserve energy supplies. In fact, in animal studies, semi-starved animals maintained nearly the same fat to muscle ratio as their well-fed litter mates.[43,44] Even worse, when food is again available the body not only gains back all the original fat but an additonal few pounds just in case this ever happens again. Is it any wonder then that yo-yo dieting leads to obesity and a host of other problems?[42,45] The reconstruction of muscle mass after starvation, a much slower process than regaining body fat, leaves a person feeling weak and even more lethargic than before he started his diet.

All Calories Are Not Created Equal

When we eat more than our daily energy requirements (and most of us do), the extra energy is stored as fat. The human body is designed to stockpile fat very easily. This tendency is related to innate mechanisms intended to protect us against starvation or the threat of a diminished food supply. Fat cells provide extra fuel which can be utilized if necessary to sustain life. Those survival fat pounds settle on the hips, waist, thighs, upper arms and back, not to mention around organs, like the heart and kidney. Some ethnic groups, whose ancestors repeatedly suffered from famines, are especially efficient in energy storage. These include the Pima tribe[48] in the United States, the Aborigines of Australia,[49] and many of those of African descent.[41]

Fats are very readily converted to pounds. Carbohydrates and proteins require more complicated digestive processes to convert and store their energy than fat does. Calories from carbohydrates and proteins are usually burned and thrown off as heat (thermogenesis). Naturally, overeating proteins and carbohydrates can result in weight gain, however the body has to work harder to convert these nutrients to fat stores. It takes 20 to 25 percent of the energy in carbohydrate and protein to convert them into body fat. It only takes about 5 percent of the energy content of dietary fat to store it as body fat. Fat is also twice as energy dense (9 calories per gram) as carbohydrates or proteins (4 calories per gram) making fat at least twice as dangerous from a weight gain standpoint.[50] Blood taken from an individual soon after they have eaten a double cheeseburger, french fries and a thick milk shake will often be a milky pink color due to the infusion of fat from the digestive system. This fat circulates throughout the system until it is either burned or stored.

A Winning Combination

Most people would agree that exercise combined with a low-fat, high-fiber diet would be a winning combination for maintaining and improving health.

Exercise is important in any health maintenance program. It is especially important in weight control since the amount of energy we expend in the resting state, our Resting Metabolic Rate (RMR), is a function of our muscle mass and tone.[51,52] There is a tendency for us to lose muscle mass and gain fat pounds as we age. In part, this is due to life style changes. Instead of flying kites we fly desks! Nevertheless, our capacity to increase our muscle mass is undiminished with age.[53] The lack of exercise rather than the abundance of candy is thought to be the primary cause of childhood obesity.[54]

Eating a low-fat, high-fiber diet will produce some weight loss even in normal weight subjects.[55] The reason for this may well be the balance between fullness and satiety.[56] It is a proven fact that we can easily eat an excess of fat before we feel full or satisfied. This is because fats are twice as energy dense (9 calories/gram) as carbohydrates or proteins (4 calories/gram). By the time we are full, we have over eaten. Increasing our fiber intake helps us feel full. (Of course expensive gastric bypass surgery is another alternative.[57]) Eating a high-fiber diet helps us to feel more than just full. Low-fat, high-fiber diets are found to lead to a general lowering of cancer rates.[58]

Though the above combination of exercise, low-fat, and high-fiber may work in theory; making the theory work in practice is quite another story. Technology works against us in some ways as evidenced by this comment a woman made about her husband's physique: "He has added 20 pounds of lap since he got his lap-top [computer]." And just try to get a low calorie meal over your lunch hour. In Feburary 1996 McDonald's, an international fast food franchise, announced that it would be dropping its five-year experiment with the low-fat McLean burger (12 grams of fat). Also gone from the menu will be the Chef's salad and the side salad. The taste of the Big Mac (35 grams of fat) has apparently won out over its McLean competition. The salads seem to be a casualty of convenience. Eating a salad in the car after a quick pickup at the drive-through can be a bit challenging.

Fortunately, state-of-the-art research in the area of weight loss has discovered that through the addition of certain supplements and nutrients, the process of decreasing the amount of fat we process in the stomach and boosting the amount of fat we burn can be expedited. For those of us who suffer from a "fat imbalance" or a condition where we store more fat than we burn, it is often a matter of life or death to lose fat in order to protect our arteries and heart.

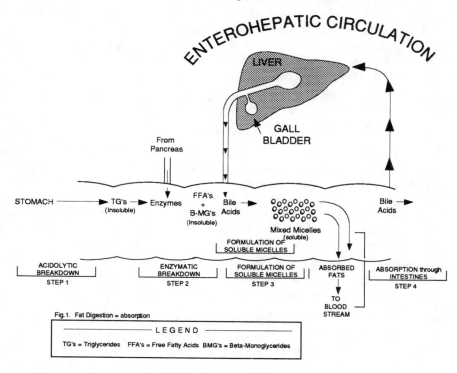

FIGURE 1. *Fat digestion and absorption*

The Secret to Weight Loss . . . An Ounce of Prevention

Most weight-reducing strategies have to confront the "after the fact" problem of burning already stored fat. Like most of our medical practices, we routinely become sick or fat and then go about the business of trying to remedy our ills. Despite Poor Richard's advice that "an ounce of prevention is worth a pound of cure," we continually eat high-fat diets, and wait until we have to pay the piper before most of us take serious action. It's much easier to prevent a fat build-up than to reverse the damage that carrying extra fat stores can cause. Going on a diet is nothing less than torture and usually means giving up all the foods we like to eat. Yet dieting seldom gets to the root cause of our excess weight which most often is that we eat too much fat, when not dieting.

The body begins to digest lipids in the stomach and intestines. The diagram in Figure 1 illustrates the steps involved in getting fat into our bloodstream.[59]

There are four steps in fat digestion: 1) acidolytic breakdown of food in the stomach; 2) enzymatic breakdown (lipolysis) of the fats (triglycerides, TGs) into fatty acids (FAs) and beta-monoglycerides (b-MGs); 3) formation of soluble mixed micelles with bile acids; and 4) absorption through the intestines. If we could tie up excess fat before it was absorbed, we could spare our physiological systems the stress of having to deal with that fat. Ideally then, what we need is a substance that prevents fat absorption.

CHITOSAN: The Fiber that Binds Fat

Overview

Chitosan is a natural product that inhibits fat absorption. It has the potential to revolutionize the process of losing weight and by so doing, reduce the incidence of some of the most devastating Western diseases we face today. Chitosan is indigestable and non-absorbable. Fats bound to chitosan become non-absorbable thereby negating their caloric value. Chitosan-bound fat leaves the intestinal tract having never entered the bloodstream. Chitosan is remarkable in that it has the abilty to absorb an average of 4 to 5 times its weight in fat.[60]

The same features that allow chitosan to bind fats endow it with many other valuable properties that work to promote health and prevent disease. Chitosan is a remarkable substance whose time has come.

Chitosan: A Brief History

Chitin, the precursor to Chitosan, was first discovered in mushrooms by the French professor Henri Braconnot in 1811.[61] In the 1820's chitin was also isolated from insects.[62] Chitin is an extremely long chain of N-acetyl-D-glucoseamine units. Chitin is the most abundant natural fiber next to cellulose and is similar to cellulose in many respects. The most abundant source of chitin is in the shells of shellfish such as crab and shrimp. The worldwide shellfish harvest is estimated to be able to supply 50,000 tons of chitin annually.[63] The harvest in the United States alone could produce over 15,000 tons of chitin each year.[64] Chitin has a wide range of uses but that is the subject of another book.

Chitosan was discovered in 1859 by Professor C. Rouget.[65] It is made by cooking chitin in alkali, much like the process for making natural soaps. After it is cooked the links of the chitosan chain are made up of glucosamine units. Each glucosamine unit contains a free amino group. These groups can take on a positive charge which gives chitosan its amazing properties. The stucture of chitosan is represented schematically in Figure 2.

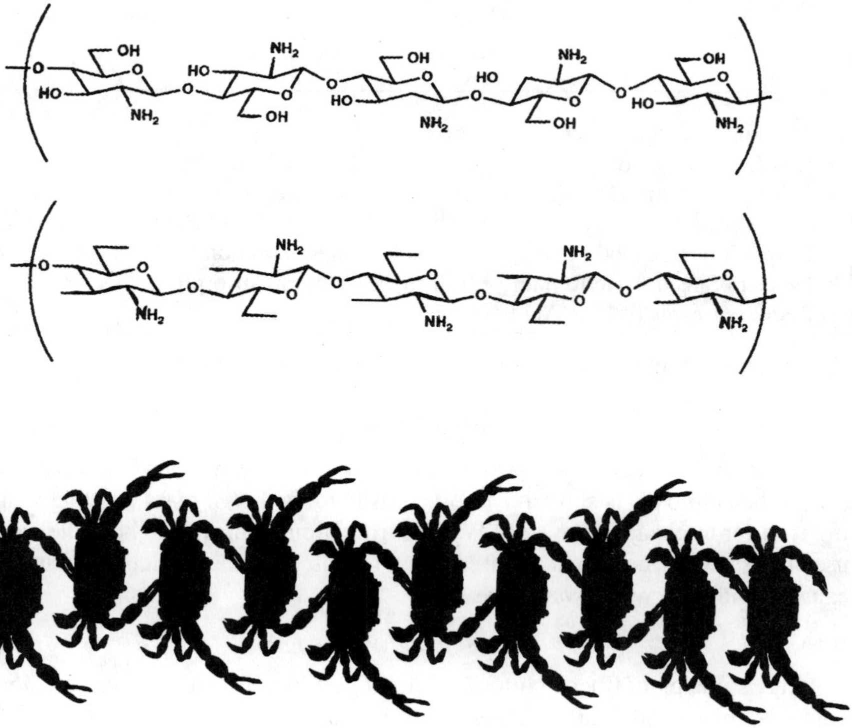

FIGURE 2. *a) Chitosan full structure*
b) Abbreviated Chitosan structure
c) Fanciful "crab oligomer" Chitosan structure showing functional claw

Research on the uses of chitin and Chitosan flourished in the 1930s and early 1940s but the rise of synthetic fibers, like the rise of synthetic medicines, overshadowed the interest in natural products. Interest in natural products, including chitin and chitosan, gained a resurgence in the 1970s and has continued to expand ever since.

Uses of Chitosan

Some of Chitosan's major uses—both Industrial and Health and Nutritional—are listed in Tables 5 and 6.

• Waste Water Purification	• Stabilizing Oil Spills
• Stabilizing Fats in Food Preparation	• Antibacterial Protection for Seeds
• Flavor Stabilizer	• Stabilizes Perishable Fruits/Vegetables
• Ion Exchange Media	• Bacterial Immobilizer
• Cosmetic and Shampoo Additive	• Tableting Excipient
• Absorbant for Heavy Metal Removal	

Table 5. *Industrial Uses of Chitosan* [66-75]

• Absorbs and Binds Fat	• Promotes Weight Loss
• Reduces LDL Cholesterol	• Boosts HDL Cholesterol
• Promotes Wound Healing	• Antibacterial/Anticandida/Antiviral
• Acts as Antacid	• Inhibits the Formation of Plaque/Tooth Decay
• Helps Control Blood Pressure	• Helps Dental Restoration/Recovery
• Helps to Speed Bone Repair	• Improves Calcium Absorption
• Reduces Levels of Uric Acid	

Table 6. *Health and Nutrition Uses of Chitosan* [60,66,77-107]

Water Purification

Chitosan has been used for about three decades in water purification processes.[67] When chitosan is spread over oil spills it holds the oil mass together making it easier to clean up the spill. Water purification plants throughout the world use chitosan to remove oils, grease, heavy metals, and fine particulate matter that cause turbidity in waste water streams.

Fat Binding/Weight Loss

Like some plant fibers, chitosan is not digestible; therefore it has no caloric value. No matter how much chitosan you ingest, its calorie count remains at zero. This is a very important property for any weight-loss product. Unlike plant fibers, chitosan's unique properties give it the ability to significantly bind fat, acting like a "fat sponge" in the digestive tract. Table 7 shows a comparison of chitosan and other natural fibers and their ability to inhibit fat absorption.

Under optimal conditions, Chitosan can bind an average of 4 to 5 times its weight with all the lipid aggregates tested.[60] (NOTE: This assessment was made without the addition of ascorbic acid which potentiates this action even further.[77] Studies in Helsinki have shown that individuals taking chitosan lost an average of 8 percent of their body weight in a 4-week period.[76]

Chitosan has increased oil-holding capacity over other fibers.[108] Among the

Chitosan

abundant natural fibers, chitosan is unique. This uniqueness is a result of chitosan's amino groups which make it an acid absorbing (basic) fiber. Most natural fibers are neutral or acidic. Table 7 summarizes the in vivo effects in animals of various fibers on fecal lipid excretion.

Dietary Fiber	% Fat Excreted	Dietary Fiber	%Fat Excreted
Chitosan	50.8 + 21.6	Carrageen	9.6 + 1.9
Kapok	8.3 + 1.1	Sodium Alginate	8.1 + 2.2
Pectin	7.4 + 1.9	Locust Bean	6.0 + 1.8
Guar	6.0 + 1.7	Konjak	5.2 + 0.6
Cellulose	5.1 + 2.1	Karaya	4.9 + 1.5
Acacia	4.6 + 0.9	Furcellaran	4.4 + 0.9
Chitin	4.3 + 1.0	Agar	2.8 + 0.4

TABLE 7. *Effects of Dietary Fibers on Fecal Lipid Excretion* [109,110]

As can be seen from the results listed, ingestion of chitosan resulted in 5-10 times more fat excretion than any other fiber tested. D-Glucosamine, the building block of chitosan, is not able to increase fecal fat excretion. This is due to the fact that glucosamine is about 97 percent absorbed while chitosan is non-absorbable. Fats bound to glucosamine would likely be readily absorbed along with the glucosamine. Chitosan, on the other hand, is not absorbed and therefore fats bound to chitosan can not be absorbed.

Cholesterol Control

Chitosan has the very unique ability to lower LDL cholesterol (the bad kind) while boosting HDL cholesterol (the good kind).[78] Laboratory tests performed on rats showed that "chitosan depresses serum and liver cholesterol levels in cholesterol-fed rats without affecting performance, organ weight or the nature of the feces."[79] Japanese researchers have concluded that Chitosan "appears to be an effective hypocholesterolemic agent."[80] In other words, it can effectively lower blood serum cholesterol levels with no apparent side effects. A study reported in the American Journal of Clinical Nutrition found that Chitosan is as effective in mammals as cholestryramine (a cholesterol lowering drug) in controlling blood serum cholesterol without the deleterious side effects typical of cholestryramine.[81] Chitosan decreased blood cholesterol levels by 66.2 percent.[82] It effectively lowered cholesterol absorption more than guar gum or cellulose.[83] Laboratory test results indicated that a 7.5% chitosan formula maintained adequate cholesterol levels in rats, despite a dramatic increase in the intake of cholesterol.[84]

MECHANISMS OF CHITOSAN FAT-BINDING

The exact way(s) that Chitosan prevents fat absorbtion is not fully understood but a number of experimental observations support two basic mechanisms.

The first mechanism involves the attraction of opposite charges which can be compared to the attraction of opposite magnetic poles. The second entrapment mechanism can be compared to the effect of a net. In the first mechanism the positive charges on chitosan attract the negatively charged fatty acids and bile acids binding them to the indigestible chitosan fiber.

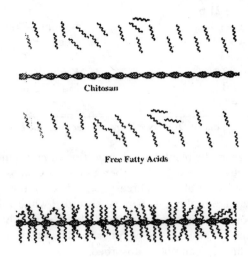

Chitosan

Free Fatty Acids

Free Fatty Acids Electrostaticly bound to Chitosan

FIGURE 3. *Magnetic mechanism used by Chitosan*

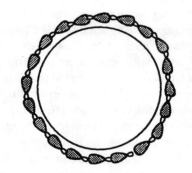

Oil Droplet Wrapped in Chitosan

FIGURE 4. *"Netting" mechanism used by Chitosan.*

This mechanism can explain why chitosan reduces LDL cholesterol levels. Our bodies make bile acids in the liver using the cholesterol from LDL. When chitosan binds bile acids it increases the rate of LDL loss thus improving the LDL to HDL ratio. If enough bile acids are bound, the fats are not solublized, which prevents their digestion and absorption.

The second mechanism (figure 2) describes a netting effect of chitosan fiber. In this model the Chitosan wraps around fat droplets and prevents their being attacked and digested by lipid enzymes. Fats unprotected by Chitosan are digested and absorbed. The "netting" mechanism has been seen to operate in vivo. [108]

Substances that Enhance the Action of Chitosan

Fibers can be likened to a tangled-up chain. Fibers must "unravel" in order for them to be of maximum benefit to us. "Unraveling" is especially critical for chitosan because each link has a hook on which to attach lipids. Chitosan can absorb an average of 4 to 5 times its weight in lipids. Reports of numbers above and below this range have also been reported and may well reflect the rate or extent of unraveling that had taken place. Fiber formulations can be prepared that unravel rapidly and swell quickly. These highly effective formulations are called superabsorbants. When certain substances are added to chitosan, its remarkable fat-binding ability can be significantly enhanced.

Ascorbic Acid

D-Ascorbic acid (erythorbic acid) and L-ascorbic acid are C-vitamins which enhance chitosan's ability to bind lipids. Combining chitosan with ascorbic acid results in even less fat absorption and greater fecal fat losses.[77,108] In one study the addition of ascorbic acid to a chitosan enriched diet increased fecal fat losses by 87 percent and decreased fat absorption by over 50 percent.[77]

Cholesterol oxides cause lesions in artery walls which predispose blood vessels to collect plaque. These dietary cholesterol oxides profoundly influence the initiation of heart disease.Free radicals can also contribute to the formation of cholesterol oxides which are even more likely to damage the heart. Cholesterol oxides have been found in deep-fried foods, powdered eggs, processed meats and in human blood itself. Consequently, taking antioxidants like ascorbic acid is vital to protect against the cellular damage this type of free radical causes.[112]

Citric Acid

In feeding experiments with animals, adding citric acid to a chitosan enriched diet resulted in a decreased feed consumption.[77] The most likely explanation for this effect is that the citric acid may be enhancing the swelling action of chitosan leading to a sense of fullness, producing satiety and appetite suppression.

Indoles

Indoles are remarkable phytochemicals which have the ability to selectively activate certain Mixed Function Oxidases (MFOs).[113] These MFO's help balance estrogen metabolism and prepare dietary toxins for elimination before they are absorbed. The presence of fiber in the intestines provides a bulk agent to carry the metabolized toxins out of the body.

Chelated Minerals

The very best approach to weight loss is to nutritionally augment food choices with nutrient supplementation. Certain biochemical compounds are essential to promoting vigor during the process of thermogenesis. Chelated minerals act to bolster, support and protect the organ systems of the body.[114,115]

For example, when fat is burned, heat and energy are released. If a lack of certain minerals exists, energy levels will drop. Minerals help to transport needed nutrients to depleted areas of the body, thereby stemming off the fatigue we so often experience after eating a fatty meal. Even more importantly, free radicals are released whenever fat is consumed and burned and the presence of chelated minerals helps to expedite the removal of these metabolites and facilitate the availability of fuel for energy.

Essential Fatty Acids

Prostaglandins control and balance many body functions. The dietary building blocks for making prostaglandins are the essential fatty acids (EFAs). The role of prostaglandins in weight loss has been extensively discussed in a recent review.[116] EFAs exert profound lipid-lowering effects. They reduce the synthesis of triglycerides and very low density lipoproteins (bad cholesterol) in the liver. EFA supplementation coupled with a low-cholesterol, low-saturated fat in diet produces a complementary effect in lowering serum lipid levels.[117]

Garcinia Cambogia (Hydroxy Citric Acid)

Garcinia Cambogia contains hydroxycitric acid (HCA). This form of citric acid inhibits the liver's ability to make fats out of carbohydrates.[118] Carbohydrates are converted to glycogen stores, not fat stores, giving the body a better energy reserve and an increase in stamina.[119]

Ephedra And Thermogenisis

Thermogenesis means "creating heat." This is one of the ways our bodies have of burning off excess calories and maintaining a constant weight.[120] This is an area of weight management research that is being intensely studied. When we repeatedly yo-yo diet or abuse ourselves by eating too much, our thermogenic ability may be reduced. Numerous animal and human studies have confirmed the benefits of ephedra and methylxanthines in inducing weight loss and restoring thermogenic responsiveness.[43,44,121]

CHITOSAN SAFETY

Chitosan is not only very useful, it is also very safe. Chitosan has been used extensively in nummerous industrial, health, and food applications.[66,71] Nevertheless, all substances when taken improperly or in gross excess can be detremental to our well-being. For example, water is normally safe when swallowed. On the other hand, breathing large amounts of water can be deadly. Similarly breathing air is relatively safe whereas intraveneous injections of air are usually fatal.

To determine the relative safety of various foods, scientists run experiments to determine the food's toxic level or LD50. Chitosan has been found to have an LD50 of over 16 grams/day/kg body weight in mice.[122] Chitosan is a fiber which expands to form a gel in the acidic environment of the stomach. The problems encountered with extremely high doses of chitosan were caused by gastric dehydration and impaction due to the expansion of the fiber.[123] To put these data in context, the authors compared Chitosan to common sugars stating "[I]t appears that chitosan is less toxic than these substances."[122] Mice are not men. For safety purposes data gathered in mice is divided by 12 to get the human equivalent.[124] The relative LD50 in humans then would be 1.33 grams/day/kg. Given that an average person weighs 150 pounds or 70 kg, this means that the toxic amount for a person would be greater than 90 grams per day. Conservatively, one could feel very confident below the 10% level, or 9 grams per day. Clinical studies have used amounts in the 3-6 grams per day range with no adverse effects. As with any fiber, a person is well advised to drink plenty of water. Changing our diets affects our colon function. Constipation or diarrehea may occur in some persons depending on their individual constitutions and on how well the Chitosan supplement was originally formulated.

Even though Chitosan is not digestible by our enzymes, it can and is degraded by soil and water microorganisms. This makes Chitosan environmentally friendly. This was recently acknowledged by the US Environmental Protection Agency when it exempted Chitosan from tolerance level testing.[68] Any breakdown of chitosan by our colon microflora would release D-glucoseamine which is itself a wonderfully beneficial nutrient for osteoarthritis sufferers.[125]

Because Chitosan can bind lipids and certain minerals, it is best to take essential fatty acid supplements, fat soluble vitamins and mineral supplements separate from Chitosan. Taking Chitosan with D- or L-ascorbic acid helps increase the amount of fat bound and decrease the loss of minerals. [77,126]

WARNINGS

YOU SHOULD NOT TAKE CHITOSAN IF YOU:

- Have Any Kind of Shellfish Allergy
- Are Pregnant or Breast-feeding

(NOTE: If you are taking medication of any kind, check with your physician before taking Chitosan. Some drugs may be bound to the Chitosan.)

The delicate nature of pregnancy and breast-feeding are always approached with additional caution. Even substances as safe as Chitosan are customarily issued with a cautionary note regarding use during these times unless overwhelmingly positive results from a huge number of well-controlled tests with pregnant subjects is available. In the case of Chitosan the potential loss of essential fatty acids (which we generally are already deficient in), fat-soluble vitamins, and certain minerals needs to be taken into consideration. Unfortunately saturated fats don't come with such a warning label.

Another caution involves allergies. Nearly all food substances will trigger allergic reactions in persons with extreme sensitivies. Since Chitosan is derived from shellfish, those persons with extreme shellfish allergies are advised to be cautious. Tests with a small number of persons with extreme shellfish allergies have not demonstrated an allergic response. This is an encouraging but very preliminary result. Reasonable and sensible consumption should always be the rule.

HOW TO TAKE CHITOSAN

The best way to take Chitosan is prior to eating a high-fat meal, which is usually lunch or dinner. Do not take with essential fatty acids, fat soluble vitamins, minerals or medications with Chitosan as their bioavailability may be inhibited. In order to avoid any type of nutrient deficiency, take your other supplements in the morning, when Chitosan is normally not used. Taking one to two grams of chitosan is adequate for most meals.

(NOTE: Whenever taking any form of fiber, drinking at least 8 glasses of water per day is highly recommended.)

SUMMARY AND CONCLUSIONS

1. **Chitosan Provides a Realistic Approach to Fat and Fiber Intake.**

Low-fat, high-fiber advocates have recommended a diet that is calorically fueled between 10 and 20 percent fat and includes 35 to 45 grams of fiber. Unfortunately, most of us, no matter how good our intentions are, will not be able to sustain this type of diet. Therefore, if we are going to face facts, a diet that reduces fat to 20-30 percent of the total caloric value and increases fiber to

20-30 grams/day is much more realistic and will help significantly in controlling weight, avoiding artery disease and promoting good colon health.

Taking Chitosan prior to eating a meal can make dietary fat goals much more attainable while promoting a number of desirable health benefits. Because obesity ranks among the top ten diseases (which, by the way, are almost all related to obesity), the availability of a safe, health-promoting fat binder is desirable.

Weight control needs to be realistic and effective. Workable weight loss programs are few and far between and usually involve a life style that many of us can never incorporate. While Chitosan is not a panacea for maintaining our youthful figures, it could be a very powerful dietary complement, facilitating what might otherwise be unattainable. Lowering the amount of dietary fats we eat, exercising more, and making sure we get enough fiber seems to be the winning combination for health and longevity. Chitosan is a valuable tool to use in attaining optimal nutrition and robust health.

2. Chitosan Is an Effective Fat Binder.

While all the previously mentioned properties of Chitosan are notable, its extraordinary ability to bind fats promises to be its most valuable asset. To reiterate, getting rid of fat after it has been stored as adipose tissue is much more difficult than neutralizing its effects before it enters the blood stream. Chitosan accomplishes this formidable task by converting fat into a form that the body does not absorb and subsequently expels.

3. Chitosan Has Remarkable Value.

Any of us who occasionally eat southern fried chicken, a Big Mac, or a slice of cheesecake every once in a while can profoundly benefit from the fat binding action of Chitosan. As a fat binder, Chitosan can significantly reduce the amount of fat that enters our blood stream.

Consider the possibilities. The foods mentioned above are full of excess fat grams. If you take four capsules (1 gram) of Chitosan with ascorbic acid, which is generally recommended, the fat content of that food is dramatically lowered.

Remember the discussion on how the liver has to deal with excess fat? Chitosan decreases the liver's work load which lightens the stress put on other body organs by the presence of excess fat. In other words, Chitosan eases the metabolic processes that kick in after we eat excess fat. As far as our metabolic processes know, those fat grams may as well never have existed.

4. Why Chitosan Is Called the Fiber of the Future.

After years of fiber "hyping" most of us are well aware of the profound benefits that fiber has for human health and longevity. Fiber is considered a dieter's best friend. It has also been linked to slower rises in blood glucose which also profoundly affects how we store excess calories and when we feel hungry.

Most fibers are hydrophilic which means they repel fat and attract water. Psyllium, for example, is used for its bulk forming action. This type of fiber absorbs water and is easily passed through the intestine, helping to maintain a normal bowel function.

Chitosan is different. While it possesses many of the same benefits as plant fibers like psyllium, Chitosan is "lipophilic" meaning that it "loves fat" It is a positively charged fiber that binds to negatively charged fatty acids. A fiber that attracts fat is unique to say the least.

Simply stated:
- *Chitosan is a non-digestible dietary fiber.*
- *Chitosan binds fats.*
- *Chitosan increases the excretion of dietary fats and cholesterol.*

ENDNOTES

1 a. The Surgeon General's "Nutrition and Health Report."
   b. The Centers for Disease Control and Prevention's "National Health and Examination Survey (NHANES III)"
   c. The National Academy of Science's. Diet and Health Report: Health Promotion and Disease Objectives (DHHS Publication No. (PHS) 91-50213, Washington, DC: US Government Printing Office, 1990).
   e.   Dietary Guidelines for Americans.

2 Rolls BJ. Carbohydrates, fats, and satiety. *Am J Clin Nutr* 1995; 61(4 Suppl):960S-967S.

3 McDowell MA, Briefel RR, Alaimo K, et al. Energy and macronutrient intakes of persons ages 2 months and over in the United States: Third National Health and Nutrition Examination Survey, Phase 1:1988-91. Advance data from vital and health statistics of the Centers for Disease Control and Prevention; No. 255. Hyattsville, Maryland: National Center for Health Statistics; 1994.

4 Center for Science in the Public Interest and McDonald's Nutrition and You—A guide to Healthy Eating at McDonald's: McDonald's Corp,1991.

5 Bray GA. Appetite Control in Adults. In: Fernstrom JD, Miller GD eds. *Appetite and Body Weight Regulation.* Boca Raton: CRC Press, 1994:1-92.

6 Michnovicz JJ. *How to Reduce Your Risk of Breast Cancer.* New York: Warner Book Inc. 1994:54.

7 Carcinogens and Anticarcinogens in the Human Diet. National Research Council Report, National Academy of Sciences, 15 Feb. 1996.

8 Van Tallie TB. Obesity: adverse effects on health and longevity. *Am J Clin Nutr* 1979:32: 2723-33.

9 Somer E, M.A. R.D. *Nutrition for Women.* New York: Henry Hold and Company, 1993:273.

10 Swaneck GE, Fishman J. Covalent binding of the endogenous estrogen 16A-hydroxyestrone to estradiol in human breast concer cells: characterization and intranuclear localization. Proc Natl Acad Sci USA 1988:85;7831-5.

11 Colditz GA. Epidemiology of breast cancer. Findings from the nurses' health study. Cancer1993;714:1480-9.

12 Hennen WJ. Breast Cancer Risk Reduction. The effects of supplementation with dietary indoles. Unpublished report 1992.

13 Deslypere BJ. Obesity and cancer. *Metabolism* 1995;44(93):24-7.

14 Somer E, M.A. R.D. *Nutrition for Women.* New York: Henry Hold and Company, 1993:281.

15 Whittemore AS, Kolonel LN, John M. Prostate cancer in relation to diet, physical activity, and body size in blacks, whites, and Asians in the United States and Canada. J Natl Cancer Inst 1995;87(9):629-31.

16 Key T. Risk factors for prostate cancer. *Cancer Survivor* 1995;23:63-77.

17 Kondo Y, Homma Y, Aso Y, Kakizoe T. Promotional effects of two-

generation exposure to a high-fat diet on prostate carcinogenisis in ACI/Seg mice. Cancer Res 1994;54(23):6129-32.

18 Wang Y, Corr JG, Taler HT, Tao Y, Fair WR, Heston WD. Decreased growth of established human prostate LNCaP tumors in nude mice fed a low-fat diet. J Natl Cancer Inst. 1995;87(19):1456-62.

19 Nixon DW. Cancer prevention clinical trials. *In-Vivo* 1994;8(5):713-6.

20 Key T. Micronutrients and cancer aetiology: the epidmiological evidence. *Proceed Nutr Soc* 1994;53(3):605-14.

21 Gorbach SL, Goldin BR. The intestinal microflora and the colon cancer connection. *Reviews of Infectious Diseases* 1990;12(Suppl 2):S252-61.

22 Shrapnel WS, Calvert GD, Nestel PJ, Truswell AS. Diet and coronary heart disease. The National Heart Foundation of Australia. *Med J Australia.* 1995;156(Suppl):S9-S16.

23 Ellis JL, Campos-Outcalt D. Cardiovascular disease risk factors in native Americans: a literature review. *Am. J. Preventive Med* 1994;10(5):295-307.

24 DiBianco R. The changing syndrome of heart failure: an annotated review as we approach the 21st century. *J. Hypertension* 1994; 12(4 Suppl):S73-S87.

25 Van Itallie TB. Obesity: adverse effects on health and longevity. *Am J Clin Nutr* 1979;32(suppl):2723-33.

26 Kestin M, Moss R, Clifton PM, Nestel PJ. Comparative effects of three cereal brans on plasma lipids, blood pressure and glucose metabolism in mildly hyper-cholesterolemic men. *Am J Clin Nutr* 1990;52(4):661-6.

27 Story JA. Dietary fiber and lipid metabolism. In: Spiller GA, Kay RM. eds. Medical Aspects of Dietary Fiber. *Penun Medical*; New York, 1980, p.138.

28 Stein PP, Black HR. The role of diet in the genesis and treatment of hypertension. *Med. Clin. North America.* 1993;77(4):831-47.

29 Olin JW. Antihypertensive treatment in patients with peripheral vascular disease. Cleve. *Clin. J. Medicine.* 1994;61(5):337-44.

30 Tinker LF. Diabetes Mellitus—a priority health care issue for women. *J. Am. Dietetic Association.* 1994;94(9):976-85.

31 Gaspard UJ, Gottal JM, van den Brule FA. Postmenopausal changes of lipid and glucose metabolism: a review of their main aspects. *Maturitas.* 1995;21(3):71-8.

32 Coordt MC, Ruhe RC, McDonald RB. Aging and insulin secretion. *Proc. Soc. Exp. Biology and Medicine.* 1995;209(3):213-22.

33 Felber JP. From Obesity to Diabetes. Pathophysiological Considerations. *Int. Journal of Obesity* 1992;16:937-952.

34 Gillum RF. The association of body fat distribution with hypertension, hypertensive heart disease, coronary heart disease, diabetes, and cardiovascular risk factors in men and women age 18-79. *J Chronic Diseases* 1987;40:421-8.

35 Haffner SM, Stern MP, Hazuda HP, et al. Role of obesity and fat distribution in non-insulin-dependent diabetes mellits in Mexican Americans and non-Hispanic whites. *Diabetes Care* 1986;9:153-61.

36 Bonadonna RC, deFronzo RA. Glucose metabolism in obesity and type 2 diabetes. *Diabetes and Metabolism.* 1991;17(1 Pt. 2):12-35.

37 Shoemaker JK, Bonen A. Vascular actions of insulin in health and disease. Canadian *J. of Applied Physiology.* 1995;20(2):127-54.

38 Resnick LM. Ionic Basis of Hypertension, Insulin Resistaince, Vascular Disease, and Related Disorders. The Mechanism of 'Syndrome X'. Am. *J. Hypertension.* 1993;6(suppl):123S-134S.

39 Trautwein EA. Dietetic influences on the formation and prevention of cholesterol gallstones. *Z. Ernahrugswiss.* 1994;33(1):2-15.

40 Cicuttini FM, Spector TD. Osteoarthritis in the aged. Epidemiological issues and optimal management. *Drugs and Aging.* 1995;6(5):409-20.

41 Melnyk MG, Wienstein E. Preventing obesity in black women by targeting adolescents: a literature review. *J Am. Diet. Association.* 1994;94(4):536-40.

42 Robinson BE, Gjerdingen Dk, Houge DR. Obesity: a move from traditional to more patient-oriented management. *J. Am. Board of Family Practice.* 1995;8(2):99-108.

43 Dulloo AG, Miller DS. Reversal of Obesity in the Genetically Obese fa/fa Zucker Rat with an Ehpedrine/Methylxanthines Thermogenic Mixture. *J. Nutrition.* 1987;117:383-9.

44 Dulloo AG, Miller DS. The thermogenic properties of ephedrin/methylxanthine mixtures: animal studies. *Am J Clinical Nutr.* 1986;43:388-394.

45 Richelsen B. Health risks of obesity. Significance of the regional distribution of adipose tissue. Ugeskr. Laeger. 1991;153(13):908-13.

46 Lissner L, Heitmann BL. Dietary fat and obesity: Evidence from epidemiology. European *J. Clinical Nutrition.* 1995;49(2):79-90.

47 Lissner L, Heitmann BL. The dietary fat: Carbohydrate ratio in relation to body weight, *Current Opinion in Lipidology.* 1995;6(1):8-13.

48 Ravussin E. Energy metabolism in obesity. Studies in the Pima Indians. *Diabetes Care.* 1993;16(1):232-8.

49 O'Dea K. Westernisation, insulin resistance and diabetes in Australian aborigines. *Med J. Australia.* 1991;155(4):258-64.

50 Bailey C. *Fit or Fat* . Houghton Mifflen, Boston, 1991.

51 McCarty MF. Optimizing Exercise for Fat Loss. Unpublished report.

52 Weinsier RL, Schutz Y, Bracco D. Reexamination of the relationship of resting metabolic rate and fat-free mass and the the metabolically active components of fat-free mass in humans. *Am. J. Clinical Nutrition.* 1992;55(4):790-4.

53 Evans WJ. Exercise, nutrition and aging. *J. Nutrition.* 1992;122(3 suppl):796-801.

54 Schlicker SA, Borra ST, Regan C. The weight and fitness status of United States children. *Nutrition Reviews.* 1994;52(1):11-7.

55 Raben A, Jensen ND, Marckmann P, Sandstrom B and Astrup A. Spontaeous weight loss during 11 weeks' ad libitum intake of a low fat/high fiber diet in young, normal weight subjects. *Stockholm Press.* 1995;916-23.

56 Blundell JE, Cotton JR, Delargy H. Green S, Greenough A, King NA,

Chitosan

Lawton, CL. The fat paradox: fat-induced satiety signals versus high fat overconsumption. *Short Communication* 1995:832-835.

57 Reinhold RB. Late results of gastric bypass surgery for morbid obesity. *J Am Coll Nutr* 1994;13(4):307-8.

58 McCredie M, Coates M Grulich A. Cancer incidence in migrants to New South Wales (Australia) from the Middle East, 1972-1991. *Cancer Causes Control* 1994:5(5):414-21.

59 Schiff ER, Dietschy JM. Steatorrhea Associated with Disordered Bile Acid Metabolism. Am. *J. Digestive Diseases.* 1969;14(6)

60 Nauss JL , Thompson JL and Nagyvary J. The binding of micellar lipids to Chitosan. *Lipids.* 1983;18(10):714-19.

61 Braconnot H, Sue la natrue ces champignons. *Ann Chim Phys* 1811;79:265.

62 Odier A. Memoire sur la composition chemique des parties cornees des insectes. *Mem Soc Hist Nat Paris* 1823;1:29.

63 Johnson EL, Peniston QP. Utilization of shellfish waste for chitin and Chitosan production. Chp 19 In: Chemistry and Biochemistry of Marine Food Products. Martin RE, Flick GJ, Hebard CE and Ward DR (eds.) 1982. p.415-. AVI Publishing Co., Westport, CT.

64 Shahram H. Seafood waste: the potential for industrial use. *Kem Kemi* 1992;19(3),256-8.

65 Rouget C. Des substances amylacees dans le tissue des animux, specialement les Articules (Chitine). *Compt Rend* 1859;48:792.

66 Chitin: A Natural Product of the 21st Century. International Commission on Natural Health Products. 1995

67 Peniston QP and Johnson EL. Method for Treating an Aqueous Medium with Chitosan and Derivatives of Chitin to Remove an Impurity. US Patent 3,533,940. Oct. 30:1970.

68 Poly-D-Glucosamine (Chitosan); Exemption from the Requirement of a Tolerance. Federal Register. 1995;60(75):19523-4. Rules and Regulations. Environmental Protection Agency 40 CFR Part 180. April, 19, 1995.

69 Arul J. "Use of Chitosan films to retard post-harvest spoilage of fruits and vegetables," Chitin Workshop. *ICNHP*, North Carolina State University, Raleigh, NC.

70 Karlsen J, Skaugrud O. "Excipient properties of Chitosan," *Manufacturing Chemist.* 1991;62:18-9.

71 Winterowd JG, Sandford PA. Chitin and Chitosan. In: *Food Polysaccharides and their Applications.* Ed: Stephen AM. Marcel Dekker 1995.

72 Chitin Workshop. *ICNHP*, North Carolina State University, Raleigh, NC.

73 Advances in Chitin and Chitosan. Eds: CJ Brine, PA Sandford, JP Zikakis. *Elsevier Applied Science.* London. 1992.

74 *Chitin in Nature and Technology.* Eds: R Muzzarelli, C Jeuniaux, GW Gooday. Plenum Press, New York. 1986.

75 Zikakis, JP. Chitin, *Chitosan and Related Enzymes.* Academic Press,

Inc. 1984.

76 Abelin J and Lassus A. Fat binder as a weight reducer in patients with moderate obesity. *ARS Medicina*, Helsinki, Aug- October, 1994.

77 Kanauchi O, Deuchi K, Imasato Y, Shizukuishi M, Kobayashi E. Increasing effect of a Chitosan and ascorbic acid mixture on fecal dietary fat excretion. *Biosci Biotech Biochem* 1994;58(9):1617-20.

78 Maezaki Y, Tsuji K, Nakagawa Y, et al. Hypocholesterolemic effect of Chitosan in adult males. *Biosci Biotchnol Biochem*1993;57(9):1439-44.

79 Kobayashi T, Otsuka S, Yugari Y. Effect of Chitosan on serum and liver cholesterol levels in cholesterol-fed rats. *Nutritional Rep. Int.*, 1979;19(3):327-34.

80 Sugano M, Fujikawa T, Hiratsuji Y, Hasegawa Y. Hypocholesterolemic effects of Chitosan in cholesterol-fed rats. *Nutr Rep. Int.* 1978;18(5):531-7.

81 Vahouny G, Satchanandam S, Cassidy M, Lightfoot F, Furda I. Comparative effects of Chitosan and cholestryramine on lymphatic absorption of lipids in the rat. *Am J Clin Nutr*, 1983;38(2):278-84

82 Suzuki S, Suzuki M, Katayama H. Chitin and Chitosan oligomers as hypolipemics and formulations containing them. *Jpn. Kokai Tokkyo Koho* JP 63 41,422 [88,422] 22 Feb1988.

83 Ikeda I, Tomari Y, Sugano M. Interrelated effects of dietary fiber on lymphatic cholesterol and triglyceride absorption in rats. *J Nutr* 1989;119(10):1383-7.

84 LeHoux JG and Grondin F. Some effects of Chitosan on liver function in the rat. *Endocrinology*. 1993;132(3):1078-84.

85 Fradet G, Brister S, Mulder D, Lough J, Averbach BL. "Evaluation of Chitosan as a New Hemostatic Agent: In Vitro and In Vivo Experiments In *Chitin in Nature and Technology*. Eds: R Muzzarelli, C Jeuniaux, GW Gooday. Plenum Press, New York. 1986.

86 Malette W, Quigley H, Gaines R, Johnson N, Rainer WG. Chitosan A New Hemostatic. *Annals of Thorasic Surgery*. 1983;36:55.

87 Malette W, Quigley H, Adickes ED. Chitosan effect in Vascular Surgery, Tissue Culture and Tissue Regeneration. In R Muzzarelli, C Jeuniaux, GW Gooday, Eds: *Chitin in Nature and Technology*. Plenum Press, New York. 1986.

88 Okamoto Y, Tomita T, Minami S, et al. Effects of Chitosan on experimental abscess with Staphylococcus aureus in dogs. *J. Vet. Med.*, 1995;57(4):765-7.

89 Klokkevold PR, Lew DS, Ellis DG, Bertolami CN. Effect of Chitosan on lingual hemostasis in rabbits. *Journal of Oral-Maxillofac-Surg,* 1991;Aug. 49(8):858-63.

89 Surgery, Tissue Culture and Tissue Regeneration. In *Chitin in Nature and Technology*. Eds: R Muzzarelli, C Jeuniaux, GW Gooday. Plenum Press, New York. 1986.

90 Hiroshi S, Makoto K, Shoji A, Yoshikazu S. Antibacterial fiber blended with Chitosan. Sixth International Conference on Chitin and Chitosan. Sea Fisheries Institute, Gdynia, Poland. August 1994;16-19.

91 Shimai Y, Tsukuda K, Seino H. Antiacne preparations containing chitin, Chitosan or their partial degradation products. *Jpn. Kikai Tokkyo Koho JP*

Chitosan

04,288,017 [92,288,017] 13 Oct 1992.

92 Suzuki K, Okawa Y, Suzuki S, Suzuki M. Candidacidal effect of peritoneal exudate cells in mice administered with chitin or Chitosan: the role of serine protease in the mechanism of oxygen-independent candidacidal effect. *Microbiol Immunol.* 1987;31(4):375-9.

93 Sawada G, Akaha Y, Naito H, Fujita M. Synergistic food preservatives containing organic acids, Chitosan and citrus seed extracts. *Jpn, Kokai Kokkyo Koho JP* 04 27,373 [92 27,373] 30 Jan 1992.

94 Min H-K, Hatai K, Bai S. Some inhibitory effects of Chitosan on fish-pathogenic oomycete, Saprolegnia parasitic. Gyobyo Kenkyu, 1994;29(2):73-4.

95 Nelson JL, Alexander JW, Gianotti L, Chalk CL, Pyles T. The influence of dietary fiber on microbial growth in vitro and bacterial translocation after burn injury in mice. *Nutr* 1994;10(1):32-6.

96 Ochiai Y, Kanazawa Y. Chitosan as virucide. *Jpn Kokai Tokkyo Koho* 79 41,326.

97 Hillyard IW, Doczi J, Kiernan. Antacid and antiulcer properties of the polysaccharide Chitosan in the rat. Proc Soc Expl Biol Med 1964; 115:1108-1112.

98 Shibasaki K, Sano H, MatsukuboT, Takaesu Y. pH response of human dental plaque to chewing gum supplemented with low molecular Chitosan. *Bull-Tokyo-Dent-Coll,* 1994:35(2): 61-6.

99 Kato H, Okuda H. Chitosan as antihypertensive. *Jpn. Kikoi Tokyo Koho JP* 06 56,674 [94 56,674]

100 Kato H, Taguchi T. Mechanism of the rise in blood pressure by sodium chloride and decrease effect of Chitosan on blood pressure. *Baiosaiensu to Indasutori* 1993;51(12):987-8.

101 Muzzarelli R, Biagini G, Pugnaoni A, Filippini O, Baldassarre V, Castaldini C, and Rizzoli C. Reconstruction of Periodontal Tissue with Chitosan. *Biomaterials.* 1989;10:598-603.

102 Sapelli P, Baldassarre V, Muzzarelli R, Emanuelli M. Chitosan in Dentistry. In *Chitin in Nature and Technology.* Eds: R Muzzarelli, C Jeuniaux, GW Gooday. Plenum Press, New York. 1986.

103 Borah G, Scott G, Wortham K. Bone induction by Chitosan in endochrondral bones of the extremities. In *Advances in Chitin and Chitosan.* Eds: CJ Brine, PA Sandford, JP Zikakis. Elsevier Applied Science. London. 1992.

104 Ito F. Role of Chitosan as a supplementary food for osteoporosis. *Gekkan Fudo Kemikaru,* 1995;11(2):39-44.

105 Nakamura S, Yoshioka T, hamada S, Kimura I. Chitosan for enhancement of bioavailability of calcium. *Jpn. Kokai Tokkyo Koho* JP 07 194,316 [95 194,316] 01 Aug 1995.

106 Maekawa A, Wada M. Food Containing chitin or its derivatives for reduction of blood and urine uric acid. *Jpn. Kokai Tokkyo Koho JP* 03 280,852 [91 280,852], 11 Dec 1991.

107 Weisberg M, Gubner R. Compositions for oral administration comprising Chitosan and a pharmaceutically acceptable carrier. Antacid preparations for alleviating gastric hyperacidity. U.S. patent 3257275

108 Kanauchi O, Deuchi K, Imasato Y, Shizukuishi M, Kobayashi E. Mechanism for the inhibition of fat digestion by Chitosan and for the synergistic effect of ascorbate. *Biosci Biotech Biochem*1995;59(5):786-90.

109 McCausland CW. Fat Binding Properties of Chitosan as Compared to Other Dietary Fibers. *Private communication.* 24 Jan1995.

110 Deuchi K, Kanauchi O, Imasato Y, Kobayashi E. *Biosci Biotech Biochem.* 1994:58,1613-6.

111 Ebihara K, Schneeman BO. Interaction of bile acids, phospholipids, cholesterol and triglyceride with dietary fibers in the small intestine of rats. *J Nutr* 1989;119(8):1100-6.

112 Weil A, M.D. *Natural Health Natural Medicine:* Boston: Houghton Mifflin, 1990:182.

113 Chen Y-H, Riby Y, Srivastava P, Bartholomew J, Denison M, Bjeldanes L. Regualtion of CYP1A1 by indolo[3,2-b]carbazole in murine hepatoma cells. *J Biol Chem* 1995;270(38):22548-55.

114 *Intestinal Absorption of metal ions and chelates.* Ashmead HD, Graff DJ, Ashmead HH. Charles C Thomas, Springfield, IL 1985.

115 *Nutrient Interactions.* Bodwell CE, Erdman JW Jr. Marcel Dekker New York 1988.

116 Heleniak EP, Aston B. Prostaglandins, Brown Fat and Weight Loss. *Medical Hypotheses* 1989;28:13-33.

117 Connor WE, DeFrancesco CA, Connor SL. N-3 fatty acids from fish oil. Effects on plasma lipoproteins and hypertriglyceridemic patients. Ann NY *Acad Sci* 1993;683:16-34.

118 Conte AA. A non-prescription alternative in weight reduction therapy. *The Bariatrician Summer* 1993:17-19.

119 McCarty MF. Inhibition of citrate lyase may aid aerobic endurance. Unpublished manuscript.

120 Bray GA. Weight homeostasis. *Annual Rev Med* 1991;42:205-216.

121 Dulloo AG, Miller DS. The thermogenic properties of Ephedrin/Methylxanthine mixtures: Human studies. *Intl J Obesity* 986;10:467-481.

122 Arai K, Kinumaki T, Fujita, T. Bulletin Tokai Regional Fisheries Res Lab. 1968;No. 56.

123 Bough WA. *Private communication.*

124 Freidrich EJ, Gehan, EA, Rall DP, Schmidt LH, Skipper HE. *Cancer Chemotherapy Reports* 1966;50(4):219-244.

125 A Drovanti, AA Bignamini, AL Rovati. Therapeutic activity of oral glucosamine sulfate in osteoarthritis: A placebo-controlled double-blind investigation. *Clinical Therapeutics* 1980;3(4):260-272.

126 K Deuchi, O Kanauchi, M Shizukuishi, E Kobayashi. Continuous and massive intake of Chitosan affects mineral and fat-soluble vitamin status in rats fed on a high-fat diet. *Biosci. Biotech. Biochemistry.* 1995;59(7):1211-6.

127 . BesChitin W in *Chitin Wound Healing* (video), Unitika Corporation, April 1992.

APPENDIX 1. ADDITIONAL DISCUSSION ON THE HEALTH AND NUTRITIONAL USES OF CHITOSAN

1. Chitosan Is A Natural Antacid

Studies have shown that Chitosan is an effective and highly safe antacid.[97] A U.S. patent has also been issued in this area.[107]

2. Antihypertensive

Some clinical studies have found that Chitosan worked as an antihypertensive agent. It lowered blood pressure in male subjects which were fed a high salt diet.[99] It also has the ability to decrease blood levels of chloride, which decreases the activity of an angiotensin converting enzyme. Angiotensin is vital to the maintenance of normal blood pressure.[100]

3. Antibacterial/Anticandida/Antiviral Properties Of Chitosan.

a) Chitosan has been effectively used to treat acne. It is able to inhibit certain bacteria which cause the inflammation associated with acne.[91]

b) Chitosan has exhibited the ability to kill candida in clinical tests involving mice due to its effect on protease action.[92]

c) When used as a food preservative, Chitosan exhibited stronger bactericidal activity than lactic acid.[93]

d) In some tests, Chitosan even demonstrated a dramatic anti- parasitic action.[94]

e) Chitosan very impressively reduced the amount of bacterial translocation which can occur after a burn injury. It is believed that by reducing the bacterial population of the colon, the potential for a life threatening infection to set in after a trauma is decreased.[95]

f) Chitosan has demonstrated the ability to kill certain viruses.[96]

- absorbs and binds fat/promotes weight loss [60,76,77]
- reduces LDL cholesterol and boosts HDL cholesterol [78-84]
- promotes wound healing [85-89]
- antibacterial/anticandida/antiviral [90-96]
- acts as an antacid [97,98]
- inhibits the formation of plaque/tooth decay [98]
- helps to control blood pressure [99,100]
- helps in dental restoration and recovery [101,102]
- helps to speed bone repair [103,104]
- improves calcium absorption [104,105]
- reduces blood levels of uric acid [106]

Table 6. *Health and Nutrition Uses of Chitosan.*

4. Wound And Ulcer Healing And Chitosan.

Tests using topical applications of Chitosan found that it promoted faster healing of wounds or abscesses that had become infected with staph infection.[88] Topical applications of Chitosan decreased coagulation time which is vital to the healing of wounds like bleeding ulcers.[89]

5. Anti-Plaque Action Of Chitosan In The Mouth.

Because of its antacid action, Chitosan increases the pH in the mouth. Chitosan also binds bacteria that cause dental plaque and subsequent tooth decay.[98]

6. Chitosan, Calcium Absorption And Bone Health.

Clinical tests have found that Chitosan enhances the bioavailability of calcium. When Chitosan is added to the diet more of the dietary calcium is absorbed.[105] The more calcium is available, the better bone quality will be. The prevention of osteoporosis depends on continual supplies of "absorbable" calcium. Chitosan has been used as a supplementary food for osteoporosis. Apparently, Chitosan activates certain macrophages which boosts the metabolism of bone and expedites the absorption of calcium from the intestine.[104]

7. Chitosan And Uric Acid.

High protein diets that come from animal sources can cause uric acid levels to rise and for some people this means a bout with gout. Chitosan has the ability to lower uric acid levels.[106]